Praise for *My Dance With Grace*

"Weldon Bradshaw has dedicated himself to making a difference in the lives of other people, to sharing his talents and passion with his community, and to leaving the world a better place than the one he inherited. He is a champion athlete and, what's more, a champion human being.

I could not be prouder that my faculty, staff, and caregiver colleagues at Virginia Commonwealth University helped heal a man who gives so much to so many people. When we talk about our commitment to human health and to catalyzing the human experience, it is with people like Weldon Bradshaw in mind."

— Michael Rao, Ph.D., President,
Virginia Commonwealth University and VCU Health System

"I have taken care of people and dealt with the ill and dying since 1980, and I have never read a more accurate or more beautiful, poetic account of defying death! Weldon's words are inspiring, and his storytelling kept me reading on and captured my very soul!"

— Dr. Robert A. Fisher, Surgical Director,
Hume-Lee Transplant Center,
Virginia Commonwealth University Medical Center

"I met Weldon Bradshaw in December of 2009 and distinctly remember an odd question at the time, as his disease seemed quite mild: 'Doc, am I going to dance at Gracie's wedding?' Three years later, on the verge of death, Weldon's last words to me before his liver transplant changed slightly, but poignantly: 'Doc, I am going to dance at Gracie's wedding.' Herein, Weldon recounts the profound change in mindset implied in the transposition of these words, which I believe helped save his life."

— Dr. R. Todd Stravitz, Medical Director,
Hume-Lee Transplant Center,
Virginia Commonwealth University Medical Center

"This book raises the stakes on the lessons that Weldon always tried to instill in me when I was his student and when I had the honor of coaching with him. After reading his story of mortality and triumph, you will see why he is still one of my most important mentors and why he is a mentor to so many others as well."

— Hon. Peter F. Farrell, Virginia House of Delegates

"Whether you are an athlete, coach, or a person that enjoys a real-life story of courage and perseverance, this book is fantastic. It will make you appreciate living life to the fullest and take nothing for granted."

— Vance Harmon, Boys Varsity Basketball Coach
Henrico High School, Richmond, Virginia

"Weldon Bradshaw hits a home run. We get a first-hand look at what a transplant patient goes through—before and after the procedure. We see how Love, Family, and Faith all help to contribute to a successful ending to a courageous battle. It is a great read for all ages!"

— Bobby Ross, former high school, college,
and professional football coach

"Weldon's story is a modern-day parable that tells of his choice to apply his everyday teaching, coaching, and spiritual philosophies to a race that gave the prize of life. He drew upon not only his inner strength and the love of his family and friends, but also the very words spoken by him to many athletes, including myself, to continue to battle through adversity and not give up. It is a compelling story told by an extraordinary man, a great coach, and a loving friend."

— Ta' Bingham Frias, Head Women's Track and Field Coach
James Madison University

"Weldon Bradshaw is the epitome of a great coach. He wants to win more than anyone, he prepares as well as anyone, he inspires and believes in his team to the end of every race and beyond, but most importantly, he understands what is important in life. Always has. The coach put up his best work as the ultimate role model and passed the test."

— Karen Doxey, Director of Athletics,
  Collegiate School, Richmond, Virginia

"Coach Bradshaw expresses in clear and concise terms the incomprehensible experience that occurs at the limits of human existence. His trial is one that remained a mystery to many of us, not only because we have not faced the reality of our mortality, but also because he is a man who bears his burdens with characteristic stoicism. He remained true to that character in his darkest hour to make it his brightest.

Coach Bradshaw conveys here the great gift he has come to understand: visceral confirmation of the lessons he has taught and coached to young men and women for four decades.

Through his own tenacity, he demonstrated that those lessons transcend running and apply to both the lightest and most dire moments of our lives.

For Weldon, it is and always has been about winning the race, regardless of the result. Weldon imparted to us—and continues to aptly discern in his own life—that *effort* and *determination* outweigh the outcomes and results toward which we are so often driven, designating the real winners in all the endeavors of our lives."

— Cabell Willis, cross country/track athlete
  Collegiate School '10, Virginia Military Institute '14

My Dance
with Grace

My Dance with Grace

Reflections on Death and Life

By Weldon Bradshaw

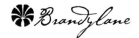

Proceeds of this book will be shared with the UNOS
Foundation and the MCV Foundation.

ISBN: 978-1-9399301-6-3

Library of Congress Control Number: 2013922515

Printed in the United States

Cover design by William Bennett.

❀ *Brandylane*
www.brandylanepublishers.com

To Emily,
my wife, my hero, the love of my life.
She kept the promise.

THE SERENITY PRAYER

God, grant me the serenity
to accept the things I cannot change;
courage to change the things I can;
and wisdom to know the difference.

Living one day at a time;
Enjoying one moment at a time;
Accepting hardships as the pathway to peace;
Taking, as He did, this sinful world
as it is, not as I would have it;
Trusting that He will make all things right
if I surrender to His Will;
That I may be reasonably happy in this life
and supremely happy with Him
Forever in the next.

Amen.

Reinhold Niebuhr

PROLOGUE

I KNOW THE COURSE BY HEART.

From the starting line, there's a slight downhill, and runners who become lost in the euphoria of the first few hundred meters quickly realize that there's enough challenging terrain remaining to suck the wind from their lungs and make their calves scream regardless of how well prepared they might be.

For years, independent school cross country teams in Virginia have run the hilly layout at Woodberry Forest School on the second Friday in November to determine state champions in four divisions.

Coaches direct their athletes' training so that they peak both physically and mentally on that day.

It's an all-or-nothing, memory-generating opportunity that those who toe the line against the backdrop of autumn beauty will replay in their heads long after their high school careers are over and they move on to the realities of life.

Before age and arthritis slowed me a decade ago, I previewed the course many times with the guys and girls whom I have coached at Collegiate School in Richmond.

As they warmed up, I reminded them of the pitfalls, the spots where they could make calculated moves, and the stretches where they could conserve energy.

I always stressed two points.

First, position yourself well, then put the hammer

down 1,100 meters from the end when you cross the paved road for the final time. The rest of the race, I explained, separates the true competitors from the pretenders. It's where championships are won or lost.

Second, never concede an advantage to the home team or any other athletes who run the course more regularly than we.

To do so signals weakness.

It reflects lack of commitment and purpose.

It provides a ready-made excuse if the outcome doesn't go our way.

While I've run the course many times, I've raced it only once.

But I wasn't on foot.

I was lying in a bed in the intensive care unit of the Virginia Commonwealth University Medical Center in the pre-dawn hours of November 14, 2012, awaiting a liver transplant that would save my life.

In my mind's eye, I was running with every fiber of my being.

There were no visible opponents or spectators, just me in shorts and T-shirt, hurtling across the rolling terrain.

A gentle, unobtrusive breeze bathed the landscape. Only the occasional, therapeutic sounds of the countryside interrupted the silence.

After passing that familiar landmark 1,100 meters from home, I negotiated a slight uphill, turned left around a directional flag, shortened my stride as I worked my way up a long, slow, devious grade, then availed myself of a gradual downhill with a long rail fence to my right.

With 700 meters to go, my legs were protesting mightily,

my heart was pounding, and my lungs felt as if they would explode.

I was on the verge of oxygen debt.

White spots were forming before my eyes.

Fatigue was overwhelming me.

Hang tough! I told myself.

Keep your eye on the prize! You know you can finish!

Find a way! Just find a way! No pain! No pain!

Ease up, and there's no tomorrow!

Literally.

Whom was I racing? Why was I racing?

I careered on. No way was I backing down.

Then the room went dark.

The anesthesia had worked its magic.

CHAPTER 1

THIS BOOK ISN'T ABOUT ME or running.

Funny, there was once a time when I thought everything in life was about me *and* running.

This book, instead, is about what I've learned from running, from competing, from coaching.

It's about all I've said to my children, grandchildren, students, athletes, and friends.

Or shown them ... hopefully.

Can you apply the lessons when the crisis is upon you?

Can you be resilient and tough when there is no alternative?

Can you be resolute when the world is unforgiving?

That is the essence of the footrace.

That is the essence of life.

During my forty-one years at Collegiate, I've offered advice, cajoled, encouraged, and attempted to summon the very best from those entrusted to my care, both in the classroom and in the athletic arena.

I've enjoyed watching them succeed.

An "A" on an exam? Excellent. A "B-" for the struggling writer who's just finding his voice? Definitely a victory, with more to come.

A championship? Great. What an enduring memory!

A personal best despite a last-place finish? Great as well, and a very special moment.

As I'd learned so clearly from my mentors, it's all about the kids. Do my job, watch them grow and flourish, help them up when they stumble, and recede into the shadows when they receive their accolades and enjoy each other's company.

It's their team, not mine.

I'm simply the director, the bus driver, the cheerleader, the equipment guy.

Now it was my turn.

Like it or not, this one *was* about me, at least for the moment.

The task was formidable.

How did I prepare for the ultimate competition?

How did I prepare for my race against death?

I couldn't let my family down.

I couldn't let my incredibly supportive friends down.

I couldn't let down the skilled physicians and nurses who had invested so much in me.

I couldn't let myself down.

I couldn't.

I wouldn't.

I absolutely wouldn't.

I DIDN'T SIDESTEP DEATH that cold November day.

Neither did I defy God's will.

The journey was challenging and occasionally unsettling and continues to be, but never has it been terrifying or even scary.

Death took no form or size or gender. It was just my

noble adversary in the race of my life.

Did God decree that I would live? I don't pretend to know, but I believe with all my heart that God granted me the strength to hold tightly to the thread of hope that remained and fight through to the very end.

Over the years, athletes have more than occasionally rolled their eyes when I've compared running to life.

Most recognize, though, that achievement in running is a short-term goal and an ephemeral experience.

Achievement in life is a long-term by-product of their effort, their work ethic, their spirit, and their abiding will to succeed.

This is their story.

This is my story.

This is truly the story of a miracle.

CHAPTER 2

IN JUNE 2009, BLOOD drawn during a routine physical exam before my right hip replacement revealed elevated liver enzyme numbers, and I was referred to Dr. R. Todd Stravitz, medical director of the Hume-Lee Transplant Center on the seventh floor of the Gateway Building at the VCU Medical Center.

A subsequent liver biopsy foreshadowed potential problems, and after further testing, Dr. Stravitz presented a "diagnosis of exclusion" of primary sclerosing cholangitis.

Exclusion? I recall asking. *You've excluded all the nasty stuff. Right?*

Little could I imagine.

Dr. Stravitz has a wonderful bedside manner, and we connected immediately. I assured him that my attitude would be great regardless of the prognosis and that I'd follow his instructions to the letter and do all within my power to assist in my treatment.

I even went so far as to promise that I'd be his absolute favorite patient ever.

He became my good friend, my advocate, and one of my guardian angels.

THE MONTHS PASSED, AND I made my quarterly visits to the clinic.

There, I saw a waiting room full of people, moving slowly, obviously sick, and discolored by jaundice, and wondered why I was even there when I could walk in unaided and actually felt pretty decent.

My answer would come soon enough.

I researched primary sclerosing cholangitis (PSC), of course, and learned that it was a progressive autoimmune disorder that would cause scarring, inflammation, and constriction in my bile ducts and ultimately prevent the toxins from leaving my liver much as a clogged drain prevents water in your sink from flowing smoothly into your sewerage system.

The disease had little "natural history," I was told, though much research was under way.

Doctors could only treat the symptoms.

If it moved slowly enough, I might even outlive PSC without incident.

If it somehow accelerated, however, it would evolve into cirrhosis, and the picture would not be pretty.

The summer after my diagnosis, I was watching a piece on television about Walter Payton, the Chicago Bears' Hall of Fame running back.

Amidst the game footage, the narrator mentioned that Payton had died at forty-five, far too young, of a rare liver disorder.

Immediately, I pulled out my BlackBerry and found a Wikipedia entry for the man called Sweetness.

He had PSC, I learned, and, by the time it was discovered, it had evolved into cholangiocarcinoma: bile duct cancer.

He was non-transplantable.

He lived just months following his diagnosis.

CHAPTER 3

OVER TIME, I BEGAN to experience significant gastrointestinal distress. It became so bad one day that Amy Rider, our school nurse, ordered me to the emergency room.

Gall bladder, the doctors speculated, but a thorough battery of tests that late spring evening in 2011 showed that all systems were in working order.

The discomfort persisted, and a subsequent colonoscopy and endoscopy revealed ulcerative colitis (UC).

My research had shown that 70 percent of people with PSC have UC.

More than likely, my PSC had triggered the UC.

In layman's terms, my body was slowly, inexorably rejecting my liver, and my liver was taking my colon with it.

Very soon, I was on a potent drug called Asacol, which muted the symptoms of UC and provided some measure of relief.

The PSC, of course, always loomed, and the upshot, I was finding, could be ugly, debilitating, and deadly.

Chapter 4

By now, I knew full well that I was playing in the big leagues. My conditions were serious, and I couldn't wish them away or tough them out, especially if my liver numbers began to rise.

Our four children, all in their thirties and spread throughout the country, were well aware that my health was declining but had no concrete details to go on. They had worried no end and encouraged me to slow down, listen to my body, and eliminate some of the responsibilities at school that led to very long workdays.

I answered that I was really fine and explained that worrying was a total waste of energy. Staying busy, I told them, kept my body energized and my mind focused squarely on the positive.

You can deny it or ignore it, you can talk a great game, but I've learned all too well that potentially catastrophic health issues are constantly in your consciousness. You wake up with them. You go to bed with them. They follow you throughout the day.

It's how you address them that determines their impact. Agonize over them, fear them, and they totally control your life. Face them with equanimity, and they will, at best, be a constant companion that enables you to reveal your true character.

Once I came to grips with the diagnoses and prognoses, I e-mailed our children.

I explained that my conditions were God-given gifts that would challenge me to be the person I had always striven to be.

For years, I reminded them, I'd worn a yellow LIVESTRONG bracelet on my left wrist to symbolize the positive qualities that I so admired in cyclist Lance Armstrong: tenacity, a steadfast refusal to quit, and a willingness to push through the limits of expectation to achieve excellence.

I also wore it, I continued, to honor those who had faced daunting, even insurmountable, obstacles and had, in the words of British poet William Ernest Henley, "neither winced nor cried aloud."

Now, I was challenging myself to measure up.

I closed my missive to the children with a heartfelt promise: *I will dance at Gracie's wedding.*

Regardless of the discomfort, the cost, or the inconvenience, I assured them, I would be there when the second oldest of my four grandchildren married.

Gracie is the only girl.

At the time, she was six years old.

CHAPTER 5

TIME ROLLED ON, AND the symptoms of PSC became more annoying, although the only ones evident to most people were my newly-acquired jaundice and fatigue. I joked about my golden tan and the yellowish hue of my eyes, but I knew full well that there was nothing funny whatsoever about steadily encroaching liver disease.

Working long hours, taking all-day Saturday road trips to track and cross country meets, and getting a decent workout—even if it involved only walking, a short stint on the exercise bike, the elliptical, or the treadmill, or light lifting—became more arduous.

I was losing muscle tone and mass, which I attempted to chalk up to advancing age, but I knew better.

On some days, I actually felt pretty good. On others, I felt as if I were slogging uphill through deep snow against a strong winter wind with a pack loaded with bricks on my back.

For most of my life, I'd been able to get by on little sleep. Now I found that it didn't take much for exhaustion to send me to the couch or the La-Z-Boy.

Eating became an adventure because I could never predict what would agree with me. Some days, pepperoni pizza hit the spot. Other times, foods as healthful as an omelet or bagel or pasta or turkey caused abdominal distress.

Soon, nothing tasted particularly good, and eating became a chore.

One day as I listlessly picked through a school lunch, a colleague who was vaguely aware of my situation asked, *Do you get any joy out of eating?*

No, not really, I replied.

It was a rare public confession that my health was slipping.

I soldiered on as best I could and never missed a day of school, a practice, an athletic competition, or a weekly freelance sports assignment for the *Richmond Times-Dispatch.*

Through all the discomfort and inconvenience, my Model for End-Stage Liver Disease (MELD) score caused no real alarm.

Tests showed that there was no malignancy, and that knowledge alone provided a great measure of solace.

During the summer of 2012, my wife Emily and I visited our children and their families in Pensacola, Boulder, and San Francisco.

We waded in the emerald water of the Gulf of Mexico and in the Pacific Ocean near the Golden Gate Bridge and absorbed the unparalleled beauty and splendor of the Rocky Mountains. We enjoyed every moment.

AirTran and Delta got us to our destinations, but the wear and tear of long-distance air travel proved more difficult than I'd ever expected as fatigue and lethargy began to enshroud my life.

Back in Richmond, I continued to consult with my physicians, but nothing in my blood work suggested immediate concern.

As the summer came to a close, however, I realized that despite the lab numbers that determined my MELD score, I was continuing to fade. Most days, I barely kept pace, but I did all that I could to maintain a smile on my face and a spring in my step. I worked from my desk as often as possible and marshaled my strength and energy as well as I could. Occasionally, I worked from home.

My sleep became more fitful and erratic. My mind often raced, not with anxiety or fear but with thoughts about my family as well as training my athletes, subjects for writing projects, and ideas to make my English class more exciting and enjoyable.

It was as if I were in a rush to do all that I could before the bottom dropped out.

The lack of rest only exacerbated my physical problems.

My energy continued to dissipate, and the egregious symptoms of PSC were becoming more obvious, although only my doctors, Emily, and I knew.

By early September, I was virtually certain that I wouldn't get through the school year unscathed, and I made certain that my affairs were in order.

I commissioned Family Electric to install a generator so Emily wouldn't be in a cold, dark condo if the power went out in the winter.

On several occasions, Emily and I had difficult and emotional conversations about the plan of action if I didn't survive.

Since arthritis overtook my hip, I had coached from a bicycle. At first, riding was therapeutic and caused no strain on my joints.

As the fall season progressed, however, the physical

demands of riding alongside even our back-of-the-pack athletes became more than I could handle. My hope was to hang tough through cross country season, which ended November 9, then enter the hospital for surgery.

It wasn't long before I was hoping just to survive the season. Period.

CHAPTER 6

By late September, my lab numbers were intensifying, and my MELD score was rising steadily. The first week in October, Dr. Stravitz filed paperwork to put me on the transplant list.

The next day, I gathered my cross country team, a delightful group of seventeen guys, many of whom had been with me season after season for several years. They knew I was ill, but they knew little more.

I explained my dilemma as objectively as possible, assured them that I'd be fine because my medical care was excellent, asked them to continue to support and encourage one another, and challenged them to perform their best at the end, whether I was a physical presence or not.

They were a rapt audience.

I could only imagine what was swirling through their heads.

Two weeks later, on Wednesday, October 17, we hosted the second of our three home meets of the season. I was so depleted that I spent most of the afternoon sitting quietly in a golf cart.

The guys listened intently to my pre-meet instructions, performed their warm-up and cool-down regimens without prompting, and ran the race with all they had while the other coaches scurried about the course and followed their progress.

Over the next two days, I supervised our long runs on the roads from my car.

My legs were too weak to pedal.

My tank was almost empty.

CHAPTER 7

ON SATURDAY, OCTOBER 20, I hit rock bottom.

After a fitful night's sleep following my final *Times-Dispatch* assignment, Emily and I joined our long-time friends Ward and Ginny Kerr, who were visiting from Southern California, for breakfast.

I then stopped by to see my dad at his apartment at Westminster Canterbury Richmond. From there I drove across town to a Collegiate alumni function to do an interview for an upcoming "Reflections," a weekly column I write for the school's website.

By the time I returned home late that afternoon, my fatigue was overwhelming. Before my hip deteriorated, I had run regularly for thirty-one years, enjoyed fifty- to sixty-mile weeks in my younger days, and completed six marathons.

Fatigue came with the territory, but what I was experiencing now made anything I had felt before seem like child's play.

I'd always considered exercise the perfect antidote for any physical problem, but the following morning, I skipped my Sunday workout at the Tuckahoe Family YMCA, a totally uncharacteristic move.

There was simply nothing left to give.

It's time, I told Emily that afternoon.

With her behind the wheel because I no longer trusted myself to drive, we headed downtown to the emergency room at the VCU Medical Center.

The greatest adventure of my life—truly an odyssey that would challenge me as never before and change me forever—had begun in earnest.

Chapter 8

In anticipation of surgery, my doctors had scheduled a battery of nine tests, which would be completed on an outpatient basis several weeks later.

They had even projected that my transplant would occur in late November or early December.

Now, the schedule was accelerated, and in the ensuing six days, I was poked, probed, prodded, invaded, scanned, and X-rayed more times than I could count to ensure that my system could endure the ravages of a transplant, which would be imminent as soon as a compatible organ became available.

Friends stopped by, and their abiding support along with flowers, cards, e-mails, and text messages reminded me that I was not making this difficult journey alone.

What I didn't understand at the time was that many of my visitors departed with a very bad feeling.

Several even mentioned much later that, based on my appearance, they feared they were bidding farewell.

I was bolstered by the frequent visits of my son David, who lives in Richmond. Earlier, he had agreed to be a living donor, to undergo surgery in which part of his liver would be implanted into me in a singular act of selflessness and love.

By the time I was admitted to the hospital, however,

before Dave could even be evaluated, my condition had deteriorated so rapidly that only a whole liver from a deceased donor would save my life.

The disease, deadly and insidious, was moving that fast.

CHAPTER 9

LATE IN THE AFTERNOON of Saturday, October 27, my doctors discharged me from the hospital and the cacophony of sounds and constant interruptions that made resting so difficult.

Thrilled to be home, I took to the guest room bed now set up in our downstairs den and eagerly awaited the call that a donor liver was available.

For nine days I remained there, reading occasionally, watching television sporadically and with little interest, and scrambling to write two "Reflections" columns before I fell completely off the face of the Earth.

Mainly, I slept.

Friends continued to call and stop by to offer encouragement.

Barty Smith, whom I've known for years, gave me a small cross containing the words "God Loves You" and the image of a dove. It hangs on a chain around my neck to this day.

Ian Rowland, a talented musician and former Collegiate runner, sent by e-mail from the University of Georgia late one night his own heartfelt recording of Neil Young's "Long May You Run."

Dave Bloor, a long-time friend and cross country counterpart at St. Catherine's School, visited with his wife

Margaret and brought a vase of flowers from his retirement party that celebrated his fifty years of coaching.

Rives and Suzanne Fleming and Charlie Blair, close friends and long-time colleagues, and George and Beth Adams, whose children had come though our distance program, checked in almost every day and provided comfort and support to both Emily and me.

The guys on my cross country team posted a heartfelt essay on the school website encouraging me to stay the course and finish the race, just as I'd encouraged them and their predecessors for thirty-five years. Their words elicited sixty-three comments, each of which inspired me to fight the good fight to the very end.

My friends at the *Times-Dispatch* and colleagues, students, and many others whom I knew from my four decades at Collegiate made clear through calls, cards, and e-mails that I was part of their families.

If I were ever tempted to lower my guard and submit to self-pity, the many random acts of kindness, positive thoughts, and prayers expressed on my behalf would have kept me smiling.

MY CONDITION CONTINUED TO deteriorate drastically, and I needed someone with me around the clock.

The plan was to get Emily to a good stopping point in her year teaching third-graders at Collegiate because we knew full well that she would soon take medical leave, as I already had, to care for me.

When Emily was at school, my sister Ann stayed at our condo, dutifully working on lesson plans and lectures for the art classes she teaches at Longwood University and checking on me regularly. Her presence and assistance were invaluable.

On Wednesday, two days before our league cross country championship, I had hoped to go briefly to school at practice time and visit with my guys, who were now being ably coached by Matthew Richardson, who headed our girls' program, and Steve Hart, who had worked with me for fourteen years.

About mid-day, as I sat at the kitchen table nibbling on a bagel, sipping a glass of tea, and halfheartedly reading the morning paper, my conversation trailed off, and my head fell forward.

When I awoke, Ann was rubbing the back of my neck and head and explaining the situation to the 911 operator.

Bleary-eyed, I dragged myself back to the den. Within a couple of minutes, paramedics from the Henrico County Fire Department arrived. I had experienced a seizure of some sort, they surmised, but I had regained my senses and assured them that I was fine.

Though they reluctantly agreed not to transport me to the hospital that day, I knew I'd experienced a serious wake-up call.

I scrapped my plans to go to school.

There was nothing I could accomplish there anyway but to alarm my guys, my coaching staff, and anyone else who might catch a glimpse of me.

Chapter 10

As my health failed, the leadership of our veterans bound the team together to create a culture—not unlike in past years—where the total exceeded the sum of the parts, and with Matthew at the helm and Steve assisting him, they couldn't have gone wrong.

A 2007 Collegiate graduate, Matthew was part of our track and cross country programs for six years. I knew by the time he was a sophomore that he'd make a great coach one day. He's instinctive, caring, and knowledgeable. As a runner in high school and at Elon University, he was quite successful, and he, like Steve, has a knack for bringing out the best in the reluctant, less talented athlete as well as those as motivated as he.

As our friendship evolved, I came to trust him completely and found it easy to turn over to him a program to which I'd given heart and soul for thirty-five years.

The guys respect him and trust his every word, but truthfully, I have no doubt they could have finished the season without a coach given their unwavering dedication to excellence and abiding support of each other and of me under the most trying conditions.

When I stepped back with three weeks remaining in the season, they had done most of their heavy training, and only the tapering and peaking phases remained. Still, the guys had to maintain their focus, no easy task when faced with a singular set of circumstances for which they had no frame of reference.

Chapter 11

THE VIRGINIA PREP LEAGUE cross country championship was contested November 2 at Panorama Farms near Charlottesville. I knew the course well, I knew the starting time, and from my bed I closed my eyes tightly and visualized the guys running every step of the rolling terrain.

It was a momentary, enjoyable respite from the challenge that was rapidly intensifying.

Early that evening after they returned, five of our seniors and Matthew visited briefly.

I congratulated them on their performances, told them how proud I was of them, thanked them for bearing with me through my physical absence and for their prayers and support, and assured them once again that while the going would be rough, I'd finish my race as strongly as they'd finished theirs.

Keep the faith, I told them. *Stay the course. Stand steady. Always stand steady.*

While I couldn't be there in person, I was with them every step of the way in spirit.

They were truly providing a bright light in an increasingly difficult interlude in my life.

CHAPTER 12

LIKE MY FIRST HOSPITAL stint, my stretch at home was mostly a blur.

Friends continued to call. Their words of support and encouragement were heartfelt and resonant. I'd spent a career trying to motivate and inspire. Now, I found myself the recipient of many gestures of kindness.

While life was moving quickly and the future appeared uncertain, I was bound and determined to hold fast until the very end.

The days came and went, and my quality time with Emily provided shelter from the rapidly gathering storm. With her abiding love and support, my spirit remained strong although my body continued to weaken.

ON ELECTION DAY, NOVEMBER 6, I returned to the transplant clinic for yet another round of lab work. The technician had trouble locating a vein since my arms had become so withered, and the nurse tending me had great difficulty finding a pulse and determining blood pressure.

My liver numbers were rising at an alarming rate, and I questioned how high they could go before a true crisis was upon us.

The cause of the rapid spike was unknown.

A distinct possibility was bile-duct cancer, and I knew

all too well that that deadly interloper would be a deal-breaker.

Noninvasive tests showed no sign of malignancy, thankfully, but I was cautioned that if surgery began and it appeared, the transplant wouldn't occur.

As we left his office that day, Dr. Stravitz commented, *We've got to get you a liver.* There was urgency and seriousness in his voice and demeanor.

He and I had developed an easy, sometimes jovial dialogue. Today, there was no joking. No joking at all.

Later that morning, Emily and I stopped by the polls at Mills Godwin High School to vote, then headed home. Sensing that the true crisis had arrived, she quickly called the clinic and told Teresa Crenshaw, my transplant coordinator, that there was no time to spare.

The results of the blood work, just in, bore out her assessment.

Around dinner time, I was admitted to the intensive care unit.

Well into the night, I watched election returns and President Obama's acceptance speech on television amidst the distracting sounds emitted by the monitors and machines next to my bed. It was the last time I would focus on anything but my health for many, many days.

When I entered the ICU, I went on a liquid diet so that if a liver became available, my system would be clear and surgery could occur quickly. For the next nine days, I was nourished by intravenous solutions and subsisted on ice chips, sips of juice, and a few peppermints.

And I never left the tight confines of my bed.

When anyone contacted me, I maintained my optimism

and commented on the superb care I was receiving. I finished each conversation with "still waiting." I said or wrote the words cheerily, I hoped, so as not to cause alarm.

I never doubted that the liver would appear, but I was making peace with the fact that my days on Earth might be coming to an end.

CHAPTER 13

MY TIME IN THE ICU, especially after darkness had fallen and my family had headed home, provided much time for reflective thought.

I found solace in the words of Rev. Buddy Childress, Rev. Bill Reeves, and Gilpin Brown, three old friends who were never far from my side and whom I often referenced as my spiritual advisors.

They guided and directed me every step of the way. We talked and laughed together. We discussed life and death. We prayed together. They were voices of reason and comfort. I clung to their every word, for they spoke the truth.

Their messages inspired and empowered me, and as the days unfolded, I convinced myself that there wasn't a worst-case scenario.

I had lived a great life with only a minimum of personal and professional rough spots, all of which now seemed trivial when cast into relief against my mounting health issues.

I truly wasn't worried and didn't want anyone else to be.

If the end were imminent, I had no regrets, no misgivings.

I could see very well how people beaten down by life and simply weary of fighting would be inclined to let go, but

I was totally unwilling to give up.

So I persevered, hoping and praying for a miracle, but reconciling myself to the fact that the outcome could be well out of my control.

Tough as it might be, I would have to accept the things I could not change.

How would I finish the race?

With poise and dignity and serenity, I hoped, and with the supreme confidence that my loved ones would be cared for and would care for one another.

Chapter 14

Perhaps my greatest inspiration during the difficult months of the fall was my longtime colleague Kevin Kelley.

In June 2012, Kevin was diagnosed with liver cancer and spent the summer receiving treatment, steeling himself for the task ahead, and preparing to return to his position as a middle school art teacher in August.

Day after day, he drove his beat-up Datsun pickup truck to school and, weak as he was, worked his magic in the classroom, just as he had for the previous twenty-five years.

His students loved him because he was kind, gentle, and intelligent and very much a kid at heart. He was an encourager and nurturer who made every student, even the less talented ones, feel that their ideas and creations were of value.

Truly, he enabled kids to realize that art is less about skill and more about self-expression.

Kevin was an accomplished sculptor, but once he entered teaching to pay the bills, he found meaning in his professional life.

He was also popular among his colleagues. He had eclectic interests and could hold forth on pretty much any topic that arose at the lunch table or in informal discussions. I hope Kevin learned as much from me over the years as I learned from him, because I learned plenty.

I saw Kevin as uncommonly tough. After all, he'd survived a year as a combat infantryman in Vietnam. He'd survived a motorcycle accident. He'd certainly survive cancer.

Or so I thought.

Throughout the fall, Kevin and I talked often and candidly about the diseases that were destroying our livers. We kept the discussions upbeat. We'd share a hospital room after transplants, keep the doctors and nurses laughing, and emerge with some great stories to tell and cool, matching scars in the shape of a Mercedes-Benz emblem.

Unfortunately, as the fall progressed, Kevin found that the cancer had spread too far and he wasn't a candidate for transplant.

He took the news of my impending surgery stoically, stared momentarily into the distance, and said, "I'm jealous."

Then, classy, selfless, and gracious as always, he wished me well as we continued the adventures of our lifetimes.

Shortly afterward, I entered the hospital, and our contact was limited to several brief phone calls.

My theme was simple: *Hang tough, Brother. There's always hope.*

In early November, Kevin went on medical leave and died on December 10 at age sixty-five.

In the time since, I've reflected often on my friend and his commitment to his students and colleagues and to Gail, his wife of forty-two years, and their two adult children.

I've reflected on his passion for art, his dedication and courage, his refusal to submit to self-pity, and his unswerving desire to play the game through to the very end.

As the months have passed, I've really missed my friend.

Amongst his family and our school family, I am not alone.

Chapter 15

On November 8, Dr. Robert A. Fisher, the surgical director of the Hume-Lee Transplant Center and a man I knew only by reputation, paid me a visit.

He introduced himself, informed me in so many words that my MELD score was skyrocketing, and then delivered a figurative forearm shiver.

If I can't transplant in a week, he said, *you'll be dead.*

He left, and I asked Emily, *Did you hear that?*

I did, she responded as she took my hand for assurance.

There was little else we could say.

I suppose I should have been overwhelmed or scared. I probably should have slipped into panic mode. But I wasn't, and I didn't.

From the outset, I had asked my doctors to be honest and forthright no matter how serious my condition became. No sugarcoating, I told them. Always tell me the truth so I'd know what I was working with.

Dr. Fisher threw down the gauntlet that day.

His declaration steeled me for the arduous task ahead. He gave me a goal that I was bound and determined to reach.

He challenged me to be courageous and steadfast and to fight for my life with every bit of emotional and spiritual resolve I could muster.

Foremost, he challenged me to be a man.

His words, harsh and blunt as they seemed at first, were perfect.

Without them, I might have cruised blithely though my final days, not fully comprehending the gravity of my situation.

Chapter 16

Our state cross country meet occurred Friday, November 9, and was contested on that same Woodberry Forest course I would run on the day my life changed forever.

Earlier that week as I quietly wondered if I would live long enough to know how our athletes performed, MileStat.com, the authoritative source for track and cross country in Virginia, ranked us tenth based on our times during the season that was quickly coming to a close.

As the championship competition unfolded, we found that our top runner, Andy Emroch, a two-time All-Prep League competitor, had injured his knee.

Like a true champion, he ran courageously over the demanding terrain with all that he had but crossed the line out of contention.

Our top eight finishers included three seniors (Teddy Nasworthy, Luke Page, and Connor Partlow), a junior (Kyle Mosman), and four freshmen (Drew McCorey, David White, John Hazelton, and William Bennett).

All the guys ran their hearts out.

We placed fifth, well ahead of the projection.

We had outperformed the performance list, exceeded expectations, lain waste to the status quo.

Five days later, with the stakes much higher, I had the

same opportunity.

I drew inspiration from my guys' spirit. I had always encouraged them. Now they were encouraging me through their words, thoughts, actions, and prayers.

I couldn't, I wouldn't, let them down.

Chapter 17

Among many other duties at school, I teach one class of seventh grade English, and after a couple of days in late August, I commented to Emily that this would be my best year of teaching ever.

The guys were energetic and respectful. I loved their vitality and work ethic. As one who enjoys seeing students improve their writing skills as much as watching runners attain lifetime bests, I was excited about the possibilities that lay ahead.

They sensed, I learned later, that I was ill. They just didn't know what was wrong, and I didn't burden them with details. The situation was unsettling enough for the older, varsity-level kids that I coach. I feared it would be too much for the twelve- and thirteen-year-olds with whom I was just beginning to bond.

In anticipation of my early exit, Dr. Kris Koebler, a retired colleague, agreed to teach my class as long as necessary.

Dutifully, she jumped in, brought expertise and professionalism to her task, and did all within her power to allay my students' fears when even she wasn't completely certain of the outcome.

I've always put my best into my teaching and coaching.

Never once did I doubt that my class and team were

receiving the same care and attention from Kris, Matthew, Steve, and the other members of our cross country staff.

CHAPTER 18

ONE BY ONE, OUR children and their families arrived.

David in Richmond checked in several times a day, often with his three-year-old son Wyatt.

Taylor, our daughter who lives in San Francisco, flew in late one night. Our other daughter, Catherine, no fan of flying, arrived from Boulder via Denver and Dallas with her almost-three-year-old son Blake.

Jay, whose home is in Pensacola, Florida, made four short trips, once with his wife Jen and children Joshua, nine, and Grace, who was then almost eight.

They put their lives and careers on hold to see and care for me and to support Emily and each other.

All booked one-way tickets.

They wondered quietly if their visits would end with a funeral or a celebration of a life restored.

My quality time with each was precious and uplifting. I gained strength from their strength.

Emily and I had met and married when her daughters and my sons were very young. Over the years, especially as they grew into adulthood, the lines of biological relationship faded. We're close to all of them. We have a special relationship with each.

If this were the end, there was joy that I'd lived life as best I could and watched our children grow into good citizens and good parents who were unfailingly loyal to their parents.

For the first time, all four of our grandchildren were together.

It was a happy, albeit brief and bittersweet, reunion.

The next time, I hoped, would be under less trying circumstances.

The youngest two would have little memory of our moments together. The older two, brother and sister, were upbeat and positive but had no idea if this was their final visit with Grandad.

It was tough duty for all, but our time was fulfilling and wonderful.

CHAPTER 19

AS TEACHERS, COACHES, AND parents, we have a golden opportunity each day to set an example. We don't even need to say much.

For me, this was one of those times.

As the week wore on, I told anyone who would listen, "I will not die in this hospital."

My assertion bolstered my family and me, but in reality I felt as if I were little more than a cocky teenager talking trash to his buddies on the blacktop during a pickup basketball game.

That was my attitude, though. It wasn't arrogance. I wasn't refuting the existence of God's plan or denying the virulence of my opponent.

It was simply my take on the final lines of Henley's "Invictus":

I am the master of my fate.
I am the captain of my soul.

Those words buoyed the spirits of Nelson Mandela during his twenty-seven-year imprisonment on Robben Island.

They were now lifting me to a level of strength and enlightenment that had once been far beyond the scope of my understanding.

If I were truly approaching "the valley of the shadow of

death," I would, in the poignant words of the Twenty-third Psalm, "fear no evil."

To follow that noble path was a validation of my faith and my upbringing.

It was a message I had to convey to my family and friends.

CHAPTER 20

ALTHOUGH I NEVER LEFT the bed, my days passed quickly.

Dr. Fisher and Dr. Stravitz visited several times, and I was tended by a legion of other highly skilled physicians and nurses who did all within their power to keep me comfortable.

They were a dedicated group, to be sure.

They exuded class and professionalism.

They were unfailingly kind, polite, and deferential, and they patiently answered my many questions.

Not once did I doubt their devotion to their calling, or, most importantly, their steadfast commitment to save my life.

BY THAT POINT, I was well aware that for me to live, someone, somewhere, would have to die.

Another family's tragedy would become my salvation. It was one of those immutable facts that engendered deep thought and even some consternation, since I'd believed all along that David would be the living donor and we'd share a singular and transformative connection.

Eventually, I came to understand that I had no say over the availability of a liver. I couldn't control the fate of others, especially from my hospital bed.

Bestowing the gift of life, I reasoned, comes from one's free will.

Before my health declined, I'd been a regular for more than thirty-five years at the Virginia Blood Service.

Long ago, my wife and I had registered as organ donors.

When we died, we would have no use for our earthly bodies, so others, we felt, should have the advantage of our commitment to health and conditioning.

For years, I had pushed my physical limits with impunity.

In my younger days, I even considered myself indestructible.

Never in my wildest dreams had I envisioned myself as an organ recipient.

CHAPTER 21

THE HOURS PASSED, BUT no compatible liver became available.

I learned later that it wasn't for lack of trying. As my MELD, which doctors cap at forty, soared upward toward fifty and I moved to the top of the transplant list, officials at the United Network for Organ Sharing (UNOS) were frantically searching for the match that would save my life.

All the while, my spirits remained good.

I was confident of a positive outcome and even joked that my liver had won Olympic gold.

I understood full well, however, that a transplant might never occur and knew that if I died, my passing would be peaceful and free of pain. I would simply close my eyes and not open them again.

Now, remember.

I'd had three years to establish my game plan and come to peace with the world. I was fighting with all my might to hold on, just as one does in the latter stages of a race that he's running more with his heart and soul than with his legs.

I'd experienced that sensation so often over the years and loved the feeling.

Never, though, had the stakes been higher.

It would have been so easy to surrender, but that, to me,

was never an option.

During the twenty-four years that I coached basketball, I'd been the one still playing to win when we were trailing by ten points with a minute to go and everyone else in the gym knew we had no chance.

I always had that last-second play designed to snatch victory from defeat.

Sometimes it worked; sometimes it didn't. But I didn't want to leave this world knowing that I hadn't covered every contingency or tried hard enough.

There was always hope.

CHAPTER 22

AS MY LIVER CONTINUED to deteriorate, my renal system began to fail as well. Only a couple of powerful jolts of dialysis kept my kidneys functioning.

The curtain was falling.

I was well aware that death was imminent. I just never accepted the fact that I would actually die.

In those final days, Buddy Childress paid me one of his many visits. He provided words of inspiration, as always, and then, holding my hand for assurance, offered a prayer.

Buddy, I said as he prepared to leave, *this is really, really hard.*

Capitulation? Absolutely not. Just a statement of fact. This was the paramount challenge of my life, but I would never, ever quit.

My life has been blessed with great family, great friends, and a great vocation and avocation.

If this were the end, I'd depart with my head held high, just as I'd seen so many friends do over the years.

If I survived this spiritual rite of passage, I'd find meaning in what came next.

CHAPTER 23

LATE IN THE EVENING on the fifth day of my allotted seven, Dr. Fisher stopped in as he made his rounds.

We thought we had a liver, he said, *but we didn't. We're still looking.*

Then he looked me squarely in the eye and said, *Mr. Bradshaw, don't give up on me.*

I told him I wouldn't, but as he turned to leave, I stopped him and countered, *Dr. Fisher, don't give up on me either.*

I'm not sure where those words came from. I wasn't challenging his authority or expertise. I meant no disrespect. I knew he was the best, but this was my way of saying that my will to survive was every bit as strong as his will to save my life.

That was all.

Simple as that.

Turns out he heard me loudly and clearly.

Turns out we already knew each other's feelings well, despite the relatively few words that had passed between us.

VIRGINIA COMMONWEALTH UNIVERSITY IS an amalgam of the Medical College of Virginia and Richmond Professional Institute.

Forty-five years post-merger, the sprawling, state-of-the-art health complex is often referenced by its original name.

During my odyssey, a friend called with the observation that MCV actually meant Miracle College of Virginia.

As time was running out, I sincerely hoped he was right.

CHAPTER 24

THE FIFTH DAY BECAME the sixth.

I was sleeping fitfully at about 2:00 A.M. when Dr. Imudia Ehanire gently awakened me.

For the past week, her kind words and compassionate manner had comforted me greatly as she made her nightly rounds.

Her presence had truly made life in the ICU manageable.

Is your phone on? she inquired.

Yes, I replied.

Expect a call within two minutes, she said.

Did they find a liver? I asked excitedly.

Her beaming smile was my answer.

At about that moment, my iPhone rang. On the other end was Teresa Crenshaw, my transplant coordinator, who, then and after, guided me gently, compassionately, and expertly through the process.

Mr. Bradshaw, she said. *Dr. Fisher has approved a liver.*

Many prayers had been answered.

Considering the moment and the sense of urgency, those were the sweetest words anyone could have spoken.

She informed me that surgery was scheduled for 10:00 A.M. She also said that Dr. Joohyun Kim would board a small jet at the Richmond International Airport around daybreak, fly to Wilmington, NC, to recover the organ, then return to Richmond.

My donor, she explained, was an eighty-four-year-old woman who had died suddenly of a stroke. She had been a pillar of her community and would be sorely missed and mourned by her family and friends.

Her liver, I was told, was in "pristine" condition.

There were risks involved and the possibility of glitches, my coordinator reminded me. But I knew full well that this was my final hope and surmised, correctly, that my medical team was essentially under-promising and would, without a doubt, over-deliver.

Thankfully, the physicians at MCV are pioneers in the transplantation of older livers—in my case, twenty years older—into younger recipients, especially those who were as sick as I was.

As I later learned, the Hume-Lee Transplant Center surgical team is the most experienced in UNOS Region 11 and has the capacity to transplant a liver more than seventy-five years old into a high MELD recipient of any age.

I also learned that my donor liver was the oldest ever transplanted anywhere, anytime, into a patient with a MELD as high as mine.

Because my doctors had the confidence and courage to attempt this delicate, risky procedure, the planets were aligning.

A miracle was truly in the making.

At that moment, I knew intuitively that I would spend the rest of my life finding meaning in the experience, and, in some small way, attempting to repay the gift.

I called Emily with the news, then Dave, then Ann, who called our dad. I called Jay, who booked the first available flight from Pensacola.

Then we contacted Charlie Blair, Collegiate's Middle School head, whom we'd asked to spread the word and be our sole conduit once the game was on so there would be no chance of misinformation.

PLAN A WAS IN action.
   It had to work.
   There was no Plan B.
   There was no second liver.

CHAPTER 25

THE ENSUING HOURS MOVED swiftly.

I signed a raft of paperwork, then turned over my computer and iPhone—my lifelines to the outside world—to Emily.

My guardian angels hurried to recover the liver and bring it to MCV as others prepared me for surgery and ultimately moved me to a staging area, my final stop before the operating room.

The energy in the large room was palpable. It was as if they were preparing for the Super Bowl and World Series all in one.

Others in my family arrived and offered comfort and consolation.

Their lives would never be the same.

They would be better, I prayed, free of worry and fear and full of a new understanding and appreciation for life.

One long, intense, unforgettable journey was ending.

Another was just beginning.

With Bill and Buddy and Gilpin at my side, I had intensified my relationship with God.

Through their words and prayers, I concluded that God was indeed giving me the strength and resolve to run this race through the finish.

If that were not enough to save my life, so be it.

Either way, I was the recipient of His amazing grace.

Chapter 26

MY CONCERN, OF COURSE, was for those I'd leave behind if I didn't survive.

Foremost, I didn't want my dad, then ninety-seven, to have to bury me. In his quiet, dignified, stoic manner, he had said little, but I knew he worried mightily.

He had grown up in the village of Rice in rural Prince Edward County, Virginia, during the pre-Depression years and had seen far too many peers die because of limited medical care and know-how.

He lost his younger sister to kidney disease when she was twenty-four.

He survived twenty months of combat and, later, occupation in the European Theater during World War II.

He has outlived most in his generation.

As a successful businessman, he has earned the abiding respect of his colleagues and competitors. The folks at Westminster Canterbury have sung his praises for years.

He's still in good health. I have no doubt he'll live to see one hundred, and I didn't want him to spend his remaining years mourning his only son.

On October 5, Emily and I had celebrated our twenty-sixth anniversary. Our yearlong courtship and marriage had been built on love and trust. We're each other's best friends and confidants. We regard each other's biological children and grandchildren as our own, not his or hers. We've worked hard at our teaching jobs.

She's supported me every step of the way, shared in my successes, comforted me through my disappointments, and put up with me when no one else would have.

She's been my soul mate, my inspiration, the love of my life. No way did I want her to endure her golden years alone.

If that were the case, however, I knew she had the steel to handle the challenge.

Throughout our ordeal, she showed uncommon strength of character and will. Despite her worries and fears, she was our linchpin, standing steady and holding our family together.

At the defining moment of her life, she was absolutely my rock. She provided love and strength and stability when, for our children, it appeared that the underpinnings of their lives were coming apart.

Mainly, she gave me a reason to live.

Our relationship with each of our children and grandchildren, as well as our daughter-in-law, is special, even unique.

Raising four children of divorce in a blended household provided many challenges.

They have different personalities, interests, talents, and temperaments.

They marched, then and now, to different drumbeats.

Over the years, they've spread throughout the country and pursued their dreams, but they still have each other's backs, and ours.

When they left the nest, we assured them that we'd

never tell them how to run their lives or raise their children, but we'd always be there for them.

This time, they were there for Emily and me.

We couldn't have asked for more.

Chapter 27

IN THE FINAL HOUR or so before I was wheeled to the operating room, I slipped quietly into a zone, much as an athlete does before a competition or a musician does before a performance.

As I vaguely discerned the flurry of activity and the voices around me, I became lost in my own world of reflection and introspection.

The images I saw were vivid.

The language I heard was of running.

There was that Shamrock 8K at Virginia Beach on a cold, brisk, forbidding Saturday morning in March 2000.

The course began at the Pavilion and took a sharp right onto Atlantic Avenue. It was originally designed to go along the boardwalk, but the organizers deemed the gale off the Atlantic Ocean too dangerous, so runners circled a series of pylons at the two-mile mark, then plunged into the northerly gusts until they reversed directions at four miles and returned home.

As I approached mile two with the wind at my back, I could see runners furiously battling the elements as they headed in the opposite direction. All appeared to be suffering. The looks on their faces and their technique spoke to their pain.

How will I handle this? I wondered. Two miles into a

brutal headwind can be daunting.

I refuse to be overwhelmed, I quickly concluded. *Instead, I'll become one with the wind.*

I taught myself a great lesson that day.

Fear the elements, fear the challenges of life, and they will surely defeat you.

Find value in the experience, and you will be invigorated and richly rewarded.

FOR SEVERAL YEARS, I dealt with an arthritic right hip, but rather than seek treatment, I attempted to out-tough an adversary that would eventually get the best of me.

When I entered the 8K that accompanied the Richmond Marathon in November 2003, I was certain that my running days were short and my racing days even shorter.

It would be the last race I'd run with any semblance of speed.

With my hip burning on every impact and the pain (which I was loath to acknowledge at the time) radiating down my leg, the adventure, perhaps ill-advised, enabled me to prove something to myself.

My downfall in 8Ks had always been the fourth mile. I could routinely hammer the first three, and adrenaline allowed me to finish strongly, but it was that stretch between miles three and four that always did me in.

This time, I wouldn't let a projected time dictate my pace. I'd run by feel and would never check my splits, I decided.

I could tell when I was giving my best. No one had to remind me. My watch wasn't the least bit necessary.

My race plan was to settle quickly into my "comfortable

hard" rhythm, maintain it through 5K, then accelerate and keep the pedal on the floor through the finish regardless of the consequences.

If my cartilage-deprived hip became too painful, I'd just focus on the crowd or the other competitors or conjure a song and play it over and over in my head.

Mainly, I'd enjoy the experience regardless of the physical demands and hold fast through the end, even if I had to crawl across the finish line.

Somewhere, I'm sure there's a record of my time, but it's really irrelevant. My plan succeeded, and I finished soaked in sweat and with a smile on my face.

My right leg throbbed mercilessly, and I limped to my car with a Gatorade in my hand and an ice bag lashed to my hip.

I'd never felt so good after a race.

Chapter 28

My thoughts in those waning hours shifted again to my parents, Ruth and Clyde Bradshaw, who have loved me despite my many weaknesses and supported me in every endeavor I've undertaken.

Four years earlier, my dad fell during his hour-long morning walk, broke his left hip, and underwent a partial replacement that kept him in the hospital for four days and the health care unit at Westminster Canterbury for another month.

Never one to sit still for long, he chafed at the confinement, but he never once complained, never placed blame, and set a sterling example for us all.

How, I thought, *could I act any differently?*

I wanted to make him proud.

We lost my mother on December 29, 2005, just two days after her ninetieth birthday. Her health had been failing, and when her time arrived, she slipped gracefully into the night with her spirit and dignity intact.

Her passing brought sadness and tears, but when I came to understand that she was at peace, I found peace.

Her Celtic music fills my iPod, her memory inspires me daily, and as my time became short, I thought of her often and reveled in my homecoming.

In my mind, as I disembarked on "the other shore," I

envisioned her waiting, radiant in beauty and with a smile crossing her face.

Son, I imagined her saying, *it's so nice to see you.*

But you're only sixty-four. Why are you here so early?

How could I tell her I hadn't tried hard enough?

How could I tell her I hadn't run with all my heart?

CHAPTER 29

YOU CAN RESEARCH LIVER disease and transplantation all you want, but you can never truly prepare for the days that follow.

My surgery occurred on a Wednesday, and the following Saturday, I awoke, finally, at 9:30 P.M. to a surreal world that I barely recognized.

Is this heaven? I wondered. *Or is it hell?*

Have I been spirited away never to see my family again?

Will life ever be the same?

I looked around tentatively.

The only familiar sight was a long yellow banner stating "Get Well Soon Mr. Bradshaw!" and signed by a host of kids and colleagues from school.

My vision was blurred and my thought process fuzzy.

Where the hell am I? I uttered, loudly enough to attract the attention of a nurse in the hallway.

Welcome back, Mr. Bradshaw, I remember her saying. *You're in intensive care at MCV. You've been here two weeks.*

You've had a liver transplant.

FOR FOUR DAYS, I had been out of touch with reality, physically restrained at times, and making irrational demands that I would never have made were I lucid.

It was a completely different persona than anyone had seen before.

My family and the attending medical team shared little except a cell phone picture with my hands and arms bound so I couldn't pull the tubes out or otherwise hurt myself or someone else.

In that picture, my eyes, viewed from deep beneath the covers, were otherworldly.

I'd read about the aftermath, but to experience it! Unbelievable!

Thankfully, I remember nothing, and my family, loyal and loving as always, stood by me, even finding some humor in the moment and understanding full well that it wasn't I, but the anesthesia, talking.

Is anyone from my family here? I asked the nurse.

In a moment, Taylor was by my side. She held my right hand and gently stroked my forehead.

It's okay, she said. You're in the same room you left earlier. Everything will be just fine.

The next day, the fog began to lift.

CHAPTER 30

WHEN I EMERGED FROM the delirium, I had been at MCV for eleven days and would remain for ten more.

By the time I was discharged on November 27, I had vowed to myself that my final act as an inpatient would be to step out of my wheelchair, walk unaided through the foyer onto East Marshall Street, get into our Hyundai Santa Fe without assistance, and begin my new life on my own terms.

It was already dark, the air was crisp and uninviting, and a gentle mist was falling on that late-autumn evening.

I'm good from here, I told the orderly as we approached the door.

Are you sure? she asked.

Quite sure, I replied. *I'm really all right.*

It was my moment of victory.

CHAPTER 31

No TRANSPLANT PATIENT, I'D been told, enjoys a smooth recovery, and I certainly haven't. Everyone reacts differently to the cocktail of medications that prevent rejection and infection and otherwise help your body adjust to a vital new organ that's the size of a football.

Further complicating the matter, I was often reminded, were the facts that my health had declined so rapidly and I was no more than a day or two from death when the surgery occurred.

In the process, my strength and energy had ebbed dramatically, and I left the hospital forty pounds below my accustomed weight.

Eating was a chore, and it was weeks before I regained my appetite. At first, the only foods that worked were yogurt and mac and cheese, which I didn't have to spend much energy chewing.

Eventually, though, my eating pattern returned to pre-PSC normal, and I slowly began to put on weight and regain some semblance of strength.

For several months post-transplant, my doctors treated me for ascites (fluid retention in my abdominal cavity), edema (swelling in my legs, ankles, and feet), and cytomegaloviral (CMV) disease that put me in the hospital for a week around Easter.

Despite regular workouts on the exercise bike, my legs remained unsteady for months. My ability to walk more than a mile or so at a time and to negotiate steps was slow to return.

Nevertheless, I had no complaints then and have none now.

You see, finally I was free and on the road to recovery, devious as that road might be.

I had survived the toughest physical and emotional challenge of my life, and the company of family and friends provided safety, security, and serenity.

Liver disease had not beaten me across the finish line.

Neither had it beaten me.

Chapter 32

So where did my approach to this lyrical, transcendent passage in my life come from?

To tell you the truth, I really don't know.

I considered it another competition, yet even the accumulation of events in which I'd participated as an athlete or coach over fifty years came nowhere close to this one.

From the outset, once I realized that major surgery was my only hope for survival, I determined there was but one way to cope with what could well be my final months.

I would be positive and proactive.

I would summon all the resolve I could muster.

I would delve into my well of faith and spirituality.

I would follow the lead of those who had dealt with health crises and do them proud.

I would set the strongest example possible for my family and friends.

I would never whine or complain.

There would be no second-guessing or plaintive cries of "Why me?"

My health challenges would neither work on my mind nor bring me down.

While my body may not survive, my spirit, I promised myself, would never, ever die.

This was purely an autoimmune issue, essentially luck of the draw, so I had no guilt feelings about the cause.

I'd just deal with PSC as best I could, use every play in my playbook, and trust God and my medical team.

If I wavered, faltered, or took my eye off the prize even for a second, no one else would ever know.

I would, though, and that realization was more than enough to sustain and motivate me.

While there was physical discomfort throughout, there was never spiritual or emotional pain, even as the clock ticked down.

I had run the best race I could.

I had come face to face with death and hadn't backed down.

In the final days, as medication numbed my body, I knew that if I were to die, I'd simply drift quietly into eternal sleep.

I'd be at peace as my mother had been seven years earlier.

The discomfort and uncertainty would be gone.

In their place would be sheer rapture.

CHAPTER 33

STRANGE AS THIS MIGHT seem, I consider my encounter with PSC and UC one of the great blessings of my life, for it challenged me to stand and deliver and summon my best when my best is needed.

Would I have felt that way if the week had come and gone, no liver had become available, and I knew I was living out my final days? I truly hope so.

The immediate crisis ended in the aftermath of my surgery. The challenge of staying healthy will be with me forever.

I'll take my medication as prescribed, listen to my body, use good judgment, get sufficient rest, eat well to sustain my weight, strength, and stamina, be patient and mindful, and avoid situations that could compromise my well-being.

It's a challenge I welcome and savor because I view life with a new understanding and a renewed relationship with God.

Throughout this incredible, unpredictable, and truly exhilarating journey, I knew I was putting each foot on the ground myself, but I never walked alone.

I knew that with the love, support, and prayers of a legion of family and friends not just in Richmond but around the country and with an expert, compassionate medical team, something magnificent had occurred.

I had stayed the course. I'd battled to the end. I'd raised my personal bar to a level that will challenge me to be like those truly courageous folks whom I've tried to honor by living strong and wearing the yellow band.

And there were times—especially as my systems were shutting down and doctors worked feverishly to keep me alive—that only two footprints appeared along the trail.

And they weren't mine.

CHAPTER 34

IN THE FOUR YEARS during which I've dealt with primary sclerosing cholangitis and ulcerative colitis, come face-to-face with my own mortality, undergone eleventh-hour liver transplant surgery, and contended with the ups and downs of the recovery process, I've received an incredible education.

Consequently, I now approach each day with a perspective that I never would have had if I had not endured the crucible and emerged as the recipient of an honest-to-goodness miracle.

My life-altering experience has provided much grist for the mill, and in the aftermath, I became even more determined to take what some might consider a negative and make it a positive.

As I've reflected on the journey, I've focused on the many valuable lessons I've learned and can share with others, so whether you're dealing with life's cheap shots or simply enjoy an inspiring story, here are several thoughts that hopefully will resonate.

BECOME AN ORGAN, TISSUE, and eye donor by signing the appropriate spot on your driver's license application or registering at www.donatelifevirginia.org (or the comparable organization in your state).

Both are legal documents.

While family permission is not required (except in the case of a minor), it's very helpful to share with your loved ones your desire to give the gift of life.

STAY IN THE MOMENT. Plan ahead certainly, but savor the small pleasures of life. Find time to read, to write, to take a leisurely walk, to think reflectively, to talk to one another.

TAKE NOTHING FOR GRANTED. Appreciate each day, the opportunities (no matter how mundane they seem), and the friendships.

YOU MIGHT TRAVEL TO dark places, but there's always a candle glowing in the distance. To view life as doom and gloom is a total waste of energy. Adversity is truly a gift that challenges you to be who you want to be.

NEVER UNDERESTIMATE THE STRENGTH and power of your family.

Likewise, never underestimate the strength and power of your extended family. Friends, at their best, share a common bond, common ideals, a common desire to care for one another.

Live long enough, and you'll minister to others and be ministered to many times over.

The abiding love, support, and encouragement of four generations of my family and my network of friends sustained me, especially as my situation became dire and the clock ticked to zero.

As a poignant reminder, many of my long-standing

competitors rallied to my side. Ben Hale, the coach at Woodberry Forest, wrote me before our state cross country meet and said, "It's like we're having a family reunion, and one of the brothers won't be there."

His words meant more to me than he could imagine. There were no Cougars or Saints or Blue Devils or Titans or Tigers. When it really counted, we were clearly teammates.

You'll learn many lessons as you travel through life. Some you'll learn the hard way. Others you'll learn more easily. The greatest lessons won't always be apparent at the moment. Chances are, though, you'll draw mightily on them when life becomes real.

Look deep within yourself for strength. My colleagues and I coach our athletes to strive for more, to exceed expectations.

Applies to life as well.

Refuse to be intimidated by obstacles that could be perceived as daunting.

Accept nothing less than your best.

Find the best in everyone. Don't harbor grudges. Respect the opinions of others, even if you disagree. Don't waste valuable energy on negative thoughts.

Approach each moment with a beginner's mind. As in a footrace, always look ahead, never behind. Learn from your mistakes and apply what you learn to new and exciting experiences and challenges.

KEEP LIFE IN PERSPECTIVE.

I was gravely ill, but many face more challenging obstacles than I did. Others have high-risk professions and callings for which they put their lives in danger every single day.

Honor them.

They are the true heroes.

EMBRACE DIVERSITY. WE SHARE our world with an eclectic mix of individuals, all vital to our community. During my time at MCV, professionals representing more nationalities, cultures, backgrounds, languages, and belief systems than I can count served me as if I were family.

TAKE CARE OF YOUR body. Be mindful of your health. Act quickly when potential problems arise. I survived for many reasons, not the least of which was the fact that my body could withstand the ravages of transplant surgery.

STAY THE COURSE. KEEP the faith, and never quit. Sometimes, you'll succeed. Sometimes you won't. Either way, you'll have no regrets.

FINALLY, ENJOY THE MIRACLE of life.

That's a cliché, I know.

Trust me, though.

It's true.

Chapter 35

My survival was nothing short of a miracle, and the promise of tomorrow is exciting beyond words.

Spreading the word through speaking and writing, counseling with individuals and families walking the same path as I, and advocating for organ donation have become my passions.

Hopefully, my experiences provide encouragement, just as the words of support, comfort, and prayer of so many others encouraged me.

So that's it.

I'm just paying forward my many blessings.

I have a story, that's for sure, but the story isn't about me at all.

It's about those whom my experiences can help.

It's about hope and inspiration.

It's about having a sense of humor, because without that vital attribute, physical and emotional pain will truly control, even destroy, your life.

It's about the power of prayer, the importance of friends and family, and the unwavering commitment of those called to medicine.

It's about applying the lessons learned and lessons taught from a long, eventful, and fulfilling lifetime.

It's about honoring my donor and her family . . . and my family.

And it's about spirituality and faith.

Without them, this ride, difficult as it was, would have been truly impossible.

A few weeks post-surgery, I commented to my friend Keith Wells, *I'm not supposed to be here.*

His response came quickly: *Maybe you are.*

So why *am* I here, typing these words, considering how close to "transitioning" I was?

I doubt I'll ever know the answer, but this I do know.

Miracles still exist in this crazy world, and for the rest of my life I will do all within my power to honor the miracle bestowed upon me that November day.

That, my friends, is my mission.

That is my challenge.

That is my sacred calling.

Epilogue

Both before my surgery and afterward, I relied heavily on wisdom I'd absorbed over the years and literary passages I'd taught and long since committed to memory.

There were the words of Henley, who wrote "Invictus" when he was in the throes of one of his myriad health crises:

Out of the night that covers me,
Black as the Pit from pole to pole,
I thank whatever gods may be
For my unconquerable soul.

In the fell clutch of circumstance
I have not winced nor cried aloud.
Under the bludgeonings of chance
My head is bloody, but unbowed.

Beyond this place of wrath and tears
Looms but the Horror of the shade,
And yet the menace of the years
Finds, and shall find, me unafraid.

It matters not how strait the gate,
How charged with punishments the scroll,
I am the master of my fate.
I am the captain of my soul.

THERE WERE PASSAGES FROM Rudyard Kipling's classic "If":

> *If you can meet with Triumph and Disaster*
> *And treat those two impostors just the same;*

> *. . . Or watch the things you gave your life to, broken,*
> *And stoop and build 'em up with worn out tools*

> *If you can force your heart and nerve and sinew*
> *To serve your turn long after they are gone,*
> *And so hold on when there is nothing in you*
> *Except the Will which says to them, "Hold on!"*

> *If you can fill the unforgiving minute*
> *With sixty seconds' worth of distance run,*
> *Yours is the Earth and everything that's in it,*
> *And—which is more—you'll be a Man, my son!*

I REFLECTED ON A familiar, thought-provoking line from Ernest Hemingway's *The Old Man and the Sea*, that Santiago, the old man, spoke with disappointment but uncommon serenity after sharks had destroyed the giant marlin, the prize of his life:

> *A man can be destroyed but not defeated.*

THERE WERE THE WORDS of Thomas Paine, the noted American political philosopher:

The harder the conflict, the more glorious the triumph.
What we obtain too cheaply, we esteem too lightly.
It is dearness only that gives everything its value.
I love the man that can smile in trouble, gather strength
from distress and grow brave by reflection.

THERE WERE VERSES FROM the Bible:

Trust in the Lord with all your heart,
and do not lean on your own understanding.
In all your ways acknowledge Him,
And He will make straight your paths.
Proverbs 3:5–6

But when the goodness and loving kindness of God our
Savior appeared, He saved us, not because of works done
by us in righteousness, but according to His own mercy, by
the washing of regeneration and renewal of the Holy Spirit,
whom He poured out on us richly through Jesus Christ our
Savior, so that being justified by His grace we might become
heirs according to the hope of eternal life.
Titus 3:4–7

For God so loved the world, that He gave His only Son,
that whoever believes in Him should not perish but have
eternal life.
John 3:16

Let us run with endurance the race that is set before us.
Hebrews 12:1

We also glory in our sufferings, because we know that suffering produces perseverance; perseverance, character; and character, hope.
Romans 5: 3–4

THERE WAS THE POEM "Do You Fear the Wind?" by Hamlin Garland:

Do you fear the force of the wind,
The slash of the rain?

Go face them and fight them,
Be savage again.

Go hungry and cold like the wolf,
Go wade like the crane:

The palms of your hand will thicken,
The skin of your cheeks will tan,

You'll grow ragged and weary and swarthy,
But you'll walk like a man!

THERE WERE THE RESPLENDENT lyrics of "You Raise Me Up" by Josh Groban:

When I am down and, oh my soul, so weary;
When troubles come and my heart burdened be;

Then, I am still and wait here in the silence,
Until you come and sit awhile with me.
You raise me up, so I can stand on mountains;
You raise me up, to walk on stormy seas;
I am strong, when I am on your shoulders;
You raise me up . . . To more than I can be.

AND THE FIRST STANZA of Neil Young's "Long May You Run":

We've been through some things together,
With trunks of memories still to come.
We found things to do in stormy weather.
Long may you run.

THERE WERE MANY RUNNING-RELATED messages that I had often imparted as advice to my athletes.

Now, in word and deed, they were imparting them to me.

Trust your preparation. You know you can finish.

Run the first part of the race with your head and the last part with your heart.

Stay as close as you can as long as you can.

Run through the finish.

The odds are only numbers. There's always hope.

Make each day, each workout, each race, your golden moment.

*Anyone can run when the wind's at his back, the
temperature's perfect, the footing is true, and the crowd is
cheering. It's what you do on the tough days when no one
is watching that makes the difference.*

*Champions concede nothing. Champions do not surrender
home-course advantage. Champions respect the weather,
the terrain, and their opponents, but they do not fear
them.*

THERE WAS THE CLASSIC quotation attributed to American
distance icon Steve Prefontaine:

To give anything less than your best is to sacrifice the gift.

THERE WERE ONE-LINE, MOTIVATIONAL messages delivered by our very wise strength and conditioning coaches to
inspire our runners as they worked in the weight room:

Tune in to Channel Excellence.
— Coach Will O'Brien

Train your compass to True North.
— Coach Adam Moss

THERE WAS THE FAMOUS declaration of former NC State
basketball coach Jim Valvano, just nine days before cancer
took his life at age forty-six:

Don't give up! Don't ever give up!

THERE WAS THE WINSTON CHURCHILL quotation inscribed on a paperweight given to me by my 2001 cross country team:

Never, Never, Never Quit

THE WORDS OF CAROLINE KEENEY, Collegiate class of 2004, have always resonated deeply with me. Caroline battled cancer most of her life. A month before she died in August 2005, she and her mother Mary-Taliaferro received the unsettling news that there was nothing more doctors could do.

As Mary-Taliaferro teared up, Caroline said simply, *Mom, stand steady!*

How could I not?

I REFLECTED ON TWO thoughts that our daughter Catherine sent me before she arrived from Colorado.

One came from the movie *Hoosiers*, when Coach Norman Dale, played by Gene Hackman, said to one of his players: *Strap, God wants you on the court.*

The other came from the poet Robert Frost and spoke volumes: *The only way around is through . . .*

SO, YOU SEE, THERE was plenty of inspiration to sustain me throughout this incredible, unforgettable passage in my life, but the most poignant message that scrolled through my head and touched my heart came not from writers or poets or coaches or athletes or philosophers or statesmen or even apostles.

It came from my then seven-year-old granddaughter.

I love you, Grandad, Grace said not in words but with

her caring smile and gentle touch as she stood with her brother by my bedside in the ICU.

You WILL dance at my wedding. I just know you will.

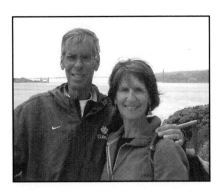

Weldon Bradshaw has worked at Collegiate School in Richmond, Virginia, since 1972, as a teacher, administrator, and coach, primarily of cross country and track.

Since 1970, he has been a freelance reporter covering mainly sports for the *Richmond News Leader*, then the *Times-Dispatch*. Since 2001, he has written a weekly column entitled "Reflections" for the Collegiate website (www.collegiate-va.org).

He and his wife Emily, who is also a teacher at Collegiate, live in western Henrico County and have four adult children and four grandchildren.

CPSIA information can be obtained at www.ICGtesting.com
Printed in the USA
BVOW07s0702290114

343207BV00001B/14/P